Smoothies for Fast Weight Loss

Smoothie Recipes, Types, & Benefits

By Katie Lenhart
Copyright © 2013

Copyright © 2013 by Katie Lenhart

ISBN-13:
978-1492253143

ISBN-10:
1492253146

All Rights Reserved. No part of this publication may be reproduced in any form or by any means, including scanning, photocopying, or otherwise without prior written permission of the copyright holder.

First Printing, 2013

Printed in the United States of America

Income Disclaimer

This book contains business strategies, marketing methods and other business advice that, regardless of my own results and experience, may not produce the same results (or any results) for you. I make absolutely no guarantee, expressed or implied, that by following the advice below you will make any money or improve current profits, as there are several factors and variables that come into play regarding any given business.

Primarily, results will depend on the nature of the product or business model, the conditions of the marketplace, the experience of the individual, and situations and elements that are beyond your control.

As with any business endeavor, you assume all risk related to investment and money based on your own discretion and at your own potential expense.

Liability Disclaimer

By reading this book, you assume all risks associated with using the advice given below, with a full understanding that you, solely, are responsible for anything that may occur as a result of putting this information into action in any way, and regardless of your interpretation of the advice.

You further agree that our company cannot be held responsible in any way for the success or failure of your business as a result of the information presented in this book. It is your responsibility to conduct your own due diligence regarding the safe and successful operation of your business if you intend to apply any of our information in any way to your business operations.

Terms of Use

You are given a non-transferable, "personal use" license to this book. You cannot distribute it or share it with other individuals.

Also, there are no resale rights or private label rights granted when purchasing this book. In other words, it's for your own personal use only.

Smoothies for Fast Weight Loss

Smoothie Recipes, Types, & Benefits

By Katie Lenhart

Table of Contents

Introduction 9
The Logic - Understanding the Basis of What Your Body Needs 11
Understanding YOU 21
Eating Today Versus Yesteryear 27
Basic Factors in Good Health 31
Types of Smoothies 33
Smoothie Benefits 39
Where Smoothies Fit In? 43
Smoothie Myths Debunked 49
Delicious Smoothie Recipes for Energy and Weight Loss 51
Final Word 57

Introduction

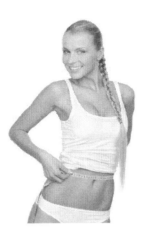

Breakfast smoothies, energy-boosting smoothies, weight-loss smoothies and healthy smoothies are just a few of the ten million different kinds of smoothies out there, all in the name of good health.

Smoothies made with wholesome ingredients are a fast and effective way to give your body the fast energy and nutrition it needs, triggering fat loss and flooding your internal systems with goodness. It's the big picture of eating healthy, exercising regularly and making sure your mental is strong, that will build your body and mind physically and mentally strong. By getting back to the basics and understanding the vitamins and minerals your body needs, you can create a plan that's going to set you on the path to energized weight loss fast. Human eating has evolved over time and today we need to be a lot more aware of what goes into our bodies. High fat processed foods loaded with dangerous toxins are packaged sweet and addictive, bombs waiting to blow in the form of disease. Something we have to UN-LEARN and stay away from.

I've studied health, nutrition and fitness for over 20 years. Through my schooling, personal experiences, and working relationships with various doctors, conventional and holistic, along with various other health professionals, I've come to understand good health on a whole new level, one that only deep experience brings. If I can pass on just one simple piece of information that helps you strengthen your health on any level, then I have succeeded in my purpose. Take it one step at a time, all eyes forward, positive and always aspiring for better. You will reach your weight loss goals and more importantly "life-health" goals if you choose to. I will help.

Smoothies are a fabulously healthy and fast way to boost weight loss, help deter disease, energize your systems, and fast-forward your progress toward looking beautiful and feeling fabulous. With your positive switch flipped and nutritious smoothie knowledge in your brain, the sky really is the limit.

The Logic - Understanding the Basis of What Your Body Needs

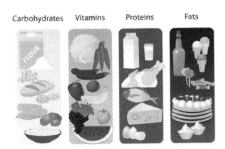

It's tough these days to always eat healthy because we live in a very stressful high-paced society drowning in convenience, including processed foods. Unfortunately, it's safe to say many of us have fallen victim to diets loaded with dangerous bad fats, tons of calories, pounds of sugar, and very little nutrition.

We seem to have forgotten that food serves a purpose. To nourish and support your bodily functions so they can provide constant energy for you to perform your daily tasks. Fumes are what we often run on because of the unhealthy foods we overstuff our bodies with, long past being full.

Did you know that by simply fueling your body with the "right" nutrients you can avert 65% of the serious diseases out there? These diseases that manifest heartache, stress, steal your quality of life and kill you prematurely.

THE MAJORITY ARE PREVENTABLE!!

Your body needs specific nutrients for growth and maintenance of energy and healthy tissues. Physical and mental stability are dependent on good nutrition.

What are nutrients?
Nutrients and the way your body processes them comprises nutrition. Your body needs both macro and micronutrients. Macronutrients like protein, carbohydrates and fat, are required in large amounts. Micronutrients are essential but less is required for optimal health.

Nonessential nutrients the body makes itself and they can also be eaten.

Essential nutrients need to come from food sources. Examples are most vitamins, a few amino acids that are protein based, and various fatty acids.

Your system is intricately balanced. Too many macronutrients can lead to obesity and related diseases that are dangerous to your healthy. Too many micronutrients may also pose toxic. For instance, if you eat a diet loaded with dangerous synthetic Trans fat, you increase your risk for developing certain kinds of disease and illness.

Macronutrients
Macronutrients make up the majority of foods you eat and are your main source of energy. They include:
Protein - including essential amino acids
Carbohydrates
Fats - including essential fatty acids
Water
You need energy for . . .
- eating and digesting food
- tissue function
- muscle use
- temperature control

- growth
- create new tissue

Oxidation is the process in which energy is released from the carbohydrates, proteins and fats you eat. Your energy requirements vary depending on your weight, height, body composition, activity level, genetics, medical condition and environment for the most part. Eating the right foods in the right amounts is one way to maximize your energy. Smoothies are a fantastic way to give your body the macronutrients it requires to function optimally.

Protein
You may have heard that proteins are the building blocks of life.
Protein is needed to . . .
* Support body tissues which stand and move, encouraging muscle contraction. Every cell in your body has protein.
* Maintain fluid balance and keep your blood healthy.
* It transports nutrients, waste and electrolytes as required throughout your body.
* Attack and neutralize disease so it doesn't invade and cause you harm, these proteins are called antibodies.
* Backup your energy sources. If you use up the energy from fats and carbohydrates, protein has no trouble stepping in.
Great protein sources are . . .
Skin-less white-meat poultry
Seafood
Eggs
Quinoa
Milk, yogurt, and various cheeses
Lean beef
Beans
Soy

Great protein sources for healthy smoothie creation are milk and yogurt to start. 2-3 servings of lean protein is recommended for most. A serving of meat is about the size of a deck of cards. For beans or yogurt 1/2 cup is a portion, and 1 cup of milk is one serving. Protein is key for building muscle and those weight training often require larger amounts of protein for the repair and building process of muscle.

Carbohydrates
Carbohydrates are comprised of starches, sugars and fiber you can get from healthy whole grains like brown rice, pasta and bread, fruits and vegetables, yogurt and milk, and essentially any food with sugar. The key here is that you fill your body full of "good" carbs or complex carbohydrates.

The two main category of carbs are:
* Complex Carbohydrates like healthy whole, beans and vegetables provide your body with LONGER LASTING energy. The key is the fiber that helps keep your blood sugars up longer and avoids those always annoying energy lows that like to hit late afternoon. Choosing to eat whole grains breads, brown rice and whole wheat pasta, along with fibrous veggies, are nutrient dense options your body needs to function optimally. Vegetable smoothies are an excellent route for giving your body a blast of energy that lasts and all the vitamins and nutrients you need to stay healthy and strong.

*Simple Carbohydrates are what you want to steer clear of for the most part, although many fruits are labeled simple carbs because they give you quick energy that doesn't last long. Of course fruits are loaded with healthy nutrients and berries in particular are comprised of healthy antioxidants that protect you from disease.

The simple carbohydrates you want to stay away from are foods like white bread, rice and pastas, processed and packaged foods like cakes, cookies, pastries and muffins. These foods are loaded with fats and sugars and will wreak havoc with your blood sugar. Immediately you will feel like you are on top of the moon and shortly after you will plummet to earth. The highs and lows of eating these fast absorbing and short lived energy foods will make you feel like you are on a roller coaster, not fun at all.

Not to mention the fact most simple carbs have little or no nutrient value. Sure they taste good and the packaging is very pretty. Fact remains they do nothing to better your health and only add to obesity, heart disease, stroke, diabetes and a whole list of other preventable and life-threatening conditions. Stay away from these convenience foods as much as you can just because your good health is important.

4-6 servings of healthy carbohydrates are what most experts recommend each day. A serving of whole grain is 1 slice, or 1/2 a bagel. Rice and pasta are examples.

Fats
Unfortunately we live in a society where fats are viewed as a bad thing. Without fat you wouldn't be able to survive. Did you know your brain is made mostly of fat? Fat helps you think straight, it protects your internal organs, gives you energy and so much more.

Fat helps your body to absorb essential vitamins like A, D, E, and K. It also gives flavor and texture to food. Without fat you can't be healthy and ultimately can't survive.

FAT DOES NOT MAKE YOU FAT!
Eating too much of anything makes you fat.

What you need to know is there are "good" and "bad" fats. Stick with the good fat and you'll do just fine.

Good Fats - In general unsaturated fats are what you want to eat. In moderation, they will help lower blood pressure and cholesterol, decreasing your risk of cardio-vascular disease and many other serious illnesses. Some healthy fats are:

- Olive, Corn and Safflower oil
- Avocado, nuts, and fatty fish like salmon

You need about 2-3 tablespoons of this vital macronutrient each day to help your body function optimally. In general we don't have to worry about not getting enough fat in our diet. We do need to focus on reducing fat and making sure we are making smart fat choices.

Bad Fats - These fats are often found in the "forbidden" foods. Tasty pastries, sweets, treats and fast food items we have programmed into our daily diet. Saturated and Trans fats are bad for us and will clog arteries, increase the risk of heart disease, diabetes, stroke and all sorts of other illness and disease that will lower our quality of life. Overloading in these bad fats is going to make you obese and this is going to open up a whole new can of worms of life-threatening factors that will eventually kill you.

Trans fats are the most dangerous because this kind of fat is chemically modified saturated fat. These fats are used in large part by mass food manufacturers because it's cheap and extends the shelf life of products tremendously. If you are eating a muffin that's good for a month, chances are it's loaded with harmful Trans fats. Unhealthy fats are only going to interfere with the intricate systems of your body. This will only cause health issues for you in time.

Some bad fats specifically are:
- Butter and lard
- Luncheon meat and poultry skin
- Full-fat dairy foods and palm oil
- Partially hydrogenated oils

By avoiding bad fats you are opening up the door for healthy living.

Water
EVERY living organism on this planet needs water to survive. You can last without food for likely a week or two, but without water you won't be around more than a few days at best.

You need water to . . .
- Regulate body temperature
- Cool your body down when it gets overheated
- Ensure electrolyte balance is maintained
- Provide body fluids for your internal systems to function
- Help keep PH levels balanced so your metabolic processes work properly

Water helps to energize and refresh you and drinking 6-8 glasses each day in essential to good health. Water hydrates your body and helps to flush harmful toxins out, toxins that will manifest overtime into disease.

Healthy and wholesome smoothies are excellent ways of giving your body the liquids it requires to function optimally. Making blended fruit smoothies with crushed ice hydrates and fuels your daily nutrient requirements in one punch. It's tasty and true.

That's the basics of macronutrients and why you need them for weight loss and good health. Next up, micronutrients.

Micronutrients
Small amounts of micronutrients are required, often because your body doesn't make them or because it needs more than it makes. Micronutrients aren't necessary for energy making but are used to make energy useable for your cells.

Vitamins are essential micronutrients made from carbon and are organic compounds
Minerals are micronutrients but the opposite, non-organic and don't have carbon.

Vitamins help other vitamins, minerals and macronutrients work better. For example, Vitamin C helps with the absorption of iron. So having citrus fruits on your steak and spinach salad makes sense, or enjoy an energizing Vitamin C Smoothie with watermelon, strawberries, cantaloupe, and low-fat yogurt works. You should have no trouble getting all the vitamins you need each day for cell reproduction, growth and energy processing by eating plenty of healthy whole grains, milk products, fresh fruits, eggs, fish, and lean meats.

Note: Only Vitamins B12, A and E are stored in the body so it's important to eat a diversified healthy diet each day. These are fat-soluble vitamins stored in fat for the most part. Overconsumption is dangerous because they can build up to toxic levels.

Water Soluble Vitamins
These are the majority and are necessary in energy processing, breaking down food for use. Examples are Vitamins B3, B2, B1, B6, B12, Folate, Vitamin C, Pantothenic Acid and Biotin.

Your body also needs plenty of fruits and vegetables for vital nutrients. They help to protect your internal systems from free radicals that look to leave you with stroke, high blood pressure, heart disease, cancer and many other preventable life-threatening conditions. Fresh berries for example are loaded with healthy antioxidants that are going to keep your immune system function strong and push illness and disease right out the back door.

Experts agree that up to 30% of breast cancers could be prevented with a healthier lifestyle and diet including regular exercise and increased fruits and vegetables.
When it comes to smoothies, fresh or frozen fruits and vegetables are the stars of the show. Endless variations of healthy nutrient dense fruits and vegetables make for energizing, tasty, metabolic boosting drinks that will help blast fat fast and leave you feeling and looking spectacular.

My Thoughts . . .
One thing you don't dictate is what your body needs to run optimally. This is already programmed into you and it's up to you to decide if you are going to fuel your body nutritiously or not. Most of us don't and end up dealing with a whole whack of preventable health issues because of this, many of them deadly over time. By choosing to make fast and nutritious smoothies a part of your diet, you are making the decision to load your body up with all of the essential macronutrients and micronutrients it requires to service you, to help trigger weight loss, and a better you mentally, physically and emotionally. As always, the choice is up to you.

Understanding YOU

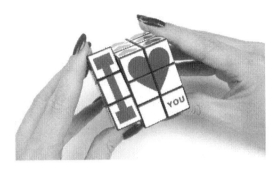

You don't need to be a nerdy scientist to know each one of us is very different, mentally, physically, emotionally and socially. Peanut butter may be your favorite protein of all, and I might be allergic to it. Exercising may be an important part of your every day and I could be challenged getting it in twice a week.

My point here is that you need to understand YOU in order to set yourself up for success. Knowing your preferences and tolerances, obstacles that may interfere with your good health, and making sure you understand "how" to register new things, is important in helping you reach your weight loss goals and so much more.

For instance, you may know that in the past you've had no trouble dropping fat. Perhaps your hurdle is in keeping it off. Maybe you aren't very active in the winter time and end up getting depressed and reverting back to your unhealthy eating habits out of boredom. That is one of your weaknesses or obstacles in weight loss, and we all have them.

By identifying this you now have the ability to make the changes necessary to break free of this pitfall and learn how to surpass this hiccup and keep your weight off for good. Maybe you need to find a new hobby or passion that is going to keep you busy in the winter months so you don't get bored and start eating junk. Making the conscious effort of side-stepping your boredom is going to give you the means to keep your hard-earned weight loss off and feel fantastic about it.

Nobody is perfect and we can only do the best we can do. Accept yourself as you are and make the verbal commitment to make the changes necessary to lose the weight you want to get healthy AND to keep it off for good, no more yo-yoing with your weight. That just stresses both your mind and body and that's not going to help you one bit.

Experimenting with delicious and nutritious smoothies, fitting them into your healthy eating strategy is only going to make losing fat and keeping it off that much easier. Making smart nutrient choices is inevitable when you are enjoying smoothies. Even if you live a crazy busy fast-paced life a smoothie will fit right in if that's what you choose.

What Interferes with Healthy Weight Loss?
The number one challenge of weight loss is the all mental. It's about accepting losing weight as a process that will have struggles. In order to be successful in weight loss you need to have a plan and a want, need, and mindset to do it. This means you're going to have to open your mind to change and focus on positivity to help push your through the challenging times. It's mind over matter here. If you really want to lose weight you can, you need to believe this if you are going to make it happen.

A few other common obstacles interfering in weight loss are . . .

CRAZY EXPECTATIONS - If you want to be successful in dropping that last 20 pounds that's literally been weighing you down, you need to flip on your logical thinking. When you are setting your goals make sure they are attainable. For instance, if you think you're going to drop 20 pounds in the first week and keep it off, you're crazy!

First, most of this weight will be water weight that's going to pile right back on the second you rehydrate yourself. Second, fat can't disappear unless you metabolize or burn it off. Sorry to burst your bubble, but this takes time and patience. There is no way to burn fat off like you would burn a matchstick, wouldn't that be nice!

A fair expectation considering you have a weight loss plan that includes making healthy food choices in moderation and exercising regularly, drinking nutritional smoothies where they fit, you should be able to drop 2-3 pounds consistently if you stick with your plan and always diversity.

It's critical you recognize your personal weight loss is influenced by a multitude of intrinsic and extrinsic factors. Fat may slough off you faster or slower one week versus the next. The idea is to persevere and stick with it. The only way you can fail in weight loss is to steer off course and stay there, or quit.

ACTION - Make sure you set realistic weight loss goals that your body and mind can physically handle. Working with a nutritionist and personal trainer are great places to start if you are beginning from square one. This investment is worth it because these professionals know what they are doing and they will help teach you to do it on your own in time. Establish a plan of action that works for you and your fat won't stand a chance.

GUILT - You are human and many people throw in the towel for weight loss because they've eaten one too many chocolate bars or went on vacation and decided to throw their healthy eating strategy, including energizing and convenient smoothies, right out the window for good.

ACTION - Let the past go. Stop beating yourself up for other fad diets that have failed. Expect to step off course from time to time because you are human. What's important is that you recognize this and get back on track pronto. Set up a strategy to help you with this. Maybe you went out with the girls and had one too many beers. So what! Fix yourself a hydrating and vitamin enriched smoothie to replace all those electrolytes you've depleted and get back to it. No harm done.

HAVING FORBIDDEN FOODS - OMG! This one will do you in every time. As humans we naturally want to do whatever we aren't supposed to, within reason anyway. By telling yourself there are specific foods you can't have, you're setting yourself up to fail in long-term weight loss. Deprivation is not a positive and eventually you will get sick and tired of the feeling, rebel and lose all of your good intended efforts.

ACTION - Understand there are no "forbidden" foods when you are trying to lose weight. YOU have the choice to eat what you want and the idea behind losing weight is to make better food choices than days past. Should you be eating a whole bag of cookies when you are looking to get slim and sexy? Nope. Although, treating yourself to a cookie on occasion is not going to steer your off course. It's all about moderation and making positive changes in your eating and lifestyle choices for life. Working tasty and vitamin enriched smoothies into your diet is one change that may distract you from all the junky foods you used to eat and steer you in the positive and energetic direction of weight loss fast and forever. It's YOUR choice.

FRUSTRATING PLATEAUS - Nobody likes a plateau and I'll be the first to say a plateau can derail a weight loss plan almost instantaneously. It's frustrating to be going through the motions, doing all the right things to lose weight and not actually see and register the results. There are plenty of strategies to avoid this and each one is easy to apply.

ACTION - Diversity is your friend when you are trying to lose weight, get healthy and make this your new normal. Weight stops coming off, because your body is used to your routine and starts to get lazy. Your mind does the same as does your physical. Without effort you aren't going to lose fat. By keeping your head and body thinking with diversity you are going to avoid frustrating plateaus.

By switching up your weights and cardio activity regularly you are going to force your body to burn more calories and your mind to stay busy. Implementing smoothies into your eating and switching them up regularly is going to boost your metabolism naturally and this means you're going to burn more fat and calories. It's a win-win situation for you.

ACCOUNTABILITY - Many people end up losing in weight loss because they don't have anyone to answer to. We seem to have no trouble disappointing ourselves, but when you bring someone else into the equation it's not so cut and dry.

ACTION - It doesn't matter who you tell, shout it out to the world if you want. The important thing here is that you make sure other people know you are losing weight and ask them to help you stick with it. Maybe you want to work with a nutritionist and each week you know you better be sticking with the program. Perhaps you will join an exercise group that will make sure you get your butt out of bed in the morning to burn fat, and that you don't go out for donuts after but have a delicious fat-burning smoothie instead. Having a support system in place will help you reach your weight loss goals and so much more.

My Thoughts . . .
Excuses just don't cut it. Either you make the decision to implement the changes necessary to lose fat and keep it off, or you don't. It's you that gets to decide if you are going to take the time to learn what delicious and nutritious smoothies suit your needs best and make sure you program them into your day to help drop fat faster and gain energy lickety-split, deter disease and boost your spirits. You control you.

Eating Today Versus Yesteryear

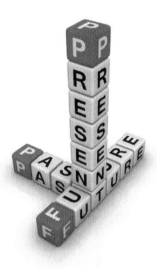

Today is a heck of a lot different when it comes to nutrition than days past. Five-hundred years ago people didn't have the convenience foods we have today. Processed and packaged unhealthy fat-laden foods with little nutritional value and a whole lot of harmful additives and preservatives. If our ancestors long past wanted to eat they had to get physical for starters. Every single thing they did for survival required intense physical demands on the body and mind, from figuring out where to best set up camp, to tracking, hunting, killing, cooking and eating dinner. Survival of the fittest was a reality then, which is definitely not the case today.

The foods available to eat were wholesome and pure, all-natural with no preservatives, pretty colors or dangerous flavorings added. Our ancestors ate only what nature provided and the closest we can come to that today is organic eating, which is more costly and not as convenient, as all the "fast" foods at our fingertips.

All we have to do when we are hungry is punch in the local pizza delivery restaurant and save up our energy to get up to answer the door when they arrive. In days past people had to put effort in to get food, so they listened to their bodies and only hunted when they were hungry.

We don't have to worry about that and because of this we often eat when we really aren't even hungry just because it's convenient. Most of us eat for emotional reasons, not physical. If our boyfriend or girlfriend dumped us we may find comfort in a big tub of triple chocolate ice cream. Hard a day at work and feeling a little tired, a hamburger and fries through the closet drive-thru is always an option. Not only are we eating calories we really don't need, but for the price of convenience we are eating all the wrong foods and missing out on giving our systems the "right" nutrients.

This quickly becomes habit and we are forever stuck in the endless cycle of pigging out on junk, dieting with deprivation, gaining the weight back and feeling depressed and frustrated with life. This cycle just keeps on going because we don't stop ourselves, smack our head against the wall a few times and set up a plan to make changes that are going to stick, ones that make sense to us and are going to help us lose fat and keep it off over time. Changes that will make us energetic and happy, stronger and more resilient to disease that will steal our life if we let it.

By sliding metabolic triggering smoothies into your regular eating plan, you're going to kick start your weight loss, give your body the nutrients in needs to function, and serve up the positive mindset to KNOW if you can "think" it you can do it.

This isn't going to be easy because as humans we are creatures of habit and by the time we realize "unhealthy" has become "us," we are already deep in routine. The first step toward change is always the hardest but if it's what you want, it will happen. Every reality begins with an idea, an idea to change your eating and lifestyle habits for the better. You are already one step closer to making this happen and you may not even realize it yet.

My Thoughts . . .
I don't want to get in too deep here, but I think it's important to recognize times are continuously changing. That's life and by first making the decision to lose fat and keep it off, you are setting yourself up for a healthy, longer, more fulfilling life. By opening your mind to using healthy smoothies to help reach your goal of losing weight fast, you're going to find this is actually going to make the journey faster and more enjoyable. Believe it!

Basic Factors in Good Health

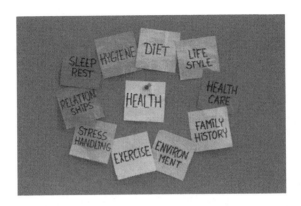

Good health is not just a one-stop-shop. There are numerous factors that determine whether or not you are or will attain good health. Encompassed here are mental, physical, emotional, social and spiritual considerations, each of which needs attention and action for ultimate good health to be reached and maintained for life. For what's good health if you don't have it long-term? Getting a little more specific, here are a few factors necessary for good overall health.

* Proper Eating
* Good Hygiene
* Regular Exercise
* Plenty of Water
* Fresh Air
* Quality sleep
* Emotional Attention
* Adequate Sunlight
* Spiritual Attention

These are the basic fundamentals in good health. By adding these up and subtracting any of the negative lifestyle habits you have, like smoking and drinking, environmental toxins from this base, you'll get your health measurement. Good health is ever-changing and a give-take relationship. By making better decisions with your fundamental health and removing the negatives of choice, you are going to improve your health and reach your goals. If your goal is to lose weight, this IS going to happen if you decide to make the changes to get there. Smoothies are a great option for helping to fuel your body optimally with few calories, trigger energy, boost immunity, trigger faster metabolism of fat and help you lose fat and keep it off for good.

My Thoughts . . .
In general if you make the decision to eat healthier, exercise your muscles and internal systems regularly, and make healthier lifestyle choices, and you stick with the program, you will drop fat and keep it off. It's all about smaller digestible steps one at a time. With each small step you take, you will get one step closer to results and it's these results that are going to keep you moving full speed ahead. Next up we're going to get down and dirty with types of smoothies available and open up the gynormous door of opportunity with fitting them into your healthy eating plan to lose weight.

Types of Smoothies

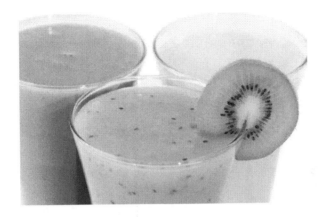

Same as cars, razors, tents and computers, smoothies come in all different shapes and sizes for all sorts of reasons. Smoothies range from sweet and rich to smooth and indulgent. The most popular are fruit smoothies, but many combine nutritious fruits and veggies for added nutritional punch. Oatmeal smoothies may hit the spot in the morning for your energetic start. Chocolate smoothies may be your afternoon mood-lifter. Believe it or not there is a smoothie for each and every eating scenario out there. Here are a few of the ones that may suit your palate:

Energy-Boosting
Energy is what makes the world go around, you too! This type of smoothie is proof that not all smoothies are created equal. This kind of smoothie truly is a beverage powerhouse. It's full of fibrous and vitamin rich fresh veggies, lean protein and plenty of other vital nutrients your body needs, that are available for quick absorption.

When you are looking for energy and weight loss it's important to take a few pointers into consideration, such as

Calories - It's just too easy to take a healthy smoothie and make it a dieter's disaster. By sticking with natural fruits to sweeten this beverage, with natural veggies and low-fat milk or yogurt for the protein and energy, and perhaps a tsp of wheat germ for some extra punch, you will get the energy boost you are looking for without the fat and calories.

Sugar - You need to be very careful here because it's really easy to overdose on the sugars in order to improve the flavor. Understand this is a "learned" preference and it can be un-learned. Again look to sweeten your energy smoothie with natural fruits and maybe a drizzle of honey if you REALLY need a little more sweet. Stay away from the extras and you will learn to enjoy your HEALTHY smoothie, minus the super sweetness.

Serving - We live in a world where everything seems to be served oversized. Don't even get me started here. It's important that you portion your energy smoothie properly and don't just make it, drink it all up and calculate that as one serving. One serving is 6-8oz. So get into the habit of divvying your beverage up and drinking accordingly, particularly when your aim is to feel energetic losing weight.

Ingredients - It's important you pay attention to what ingredients you're putting into your energy smoothie. Wholesome natural ingredients that are low in fat and high in nutrients are your aim. Throwing ice cream in a blender with a little bit of fruit and some cream to thicken it up IS NOT healthy.

Ingredients to Use:
Blueberries, raspberries, strawberries and blackberries

Nuts (almonds, macadamia nuts, Brazil nuts)
Kale and spinach
Sweet potato, banana or pineapple
Cranberries, protein powder
Low-fat milk, low-fat yogurt

Protein-Rich Breakfast
Having a smoothie in the morning is a fast way to give your body a nice dose of sustainable energy for the day. Picking a variety of nutrient-dense fruits and protein rich ingredients is going to give to a tasty start to your day that revs your engine. Remember, protein is an essential macronutrient because your body doesn't make or store it. Starting your day off with a Protein-Rich Breakfast smoothie is a great habit to get into, not to mention the fact studies show people that eat breakfast have lower body fat because their metabolism is up and running bright and early, that's one reason anyway.

Ingredients to Use . . .
Fresh berries
Ground flaxseed, oatmeal
Greek yogurt, low-fat milk
Fresh squeezed orange juice
Fresh squeezed grapefruit juice
Peanut butter

Weight-Loss
It's safe to say that most people have aren't happy with their weight, but do enjoy a diet that leaves them energized, satisfied, and a little bit thinner. Weight-Loss smoothies are a fabulous route to boosting your metabolism and helping your body burn off the excess fat stores that just aren't wanted. Green Smoothies for instance are excellent for fat burning because they are loaded with essential nutrients, packed with fiber and are low in fat.

Here are a few pointers for a uniquely satisfying Weight-Loss Smoothie:

Don't Add Fat, Knowingly or Not - Too much fat in your smoothie can trigger gas and bloating, while also interfering with your body's ability to break down the simple carbohydrates in the fruit that can lead to weight gain if overconsumption is an issue. There should be no more than a tablespoon of flaxseed or 1/4 of an avocado in one.

Aim For Little or No Sweeteners - We both know that any refined sugars added are only going to hinder your weight loss efforts. This includes adding a little white sugar that you might usually sprinkle on your strawberries. Get used to experimenting in sweetening your smoothies naturally with bananas or very ripe fruit. Dates can also be used if you really, really, really must have it sweeter. Moderation is the key, never forget it.

Avoid Store Bought Juices - This one can get you into deep trouble when trying to drop fat. Most juices are loaded with sugars and are not going to help you cut calories, boost your metabolism naturally and burn fat. It's important to get out of the habit of "thinking" adding a 1/2 cup of apple juice to your smoothie is a "healthy" move because it's not. Add an apple instead because you are getting both the natural sweetness of the apple plus fiber and essential nutrients. An apple a day does keep the doctor away!

Easy on the Added Powders - People run into trouble here because they believe that adding protein and nutrition powders is a good thing. It can be in moderation, but some of these powders are loaded with extra sugars to make them taste sweet and this will not help with weight loss. If you are adding a little bit of hemp or protein powder from time to time to boost the kick in your Weight-Loss Smoothie that's one thing. However, if you are overdoing it or choosing the wrong ones this could be the wrong move.

Ingredients to Use . . .
Bananas, berries, peaches, mangoes
Baby spinach, dates (sparingly), avocado
Flaxseed, chia seeds, nut milks, whey powder
Soy milk, almond milk, mint leaves, lemons
This book is focused on sensible weight loss and these three types of smoothies are going to support you in this. Of course, there are ten different kinds of smoothies for every color in the rainbow and you need to figure out what works for you, considering your preferences, tolerances and weight loss goals.

Smoothie Benefits

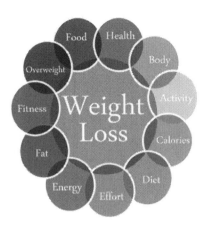

Smoothies are a fantastic way to get important vitamins and minerals into your body fast and effectively. They are tasty, healthy and nutritious and easily absorbed to start. Keep in mind a smoothie is only healthy if the ingredients you put in are healthy too. Again, moderation is the key in a balanced and healthy lifestyle and it's not hard to go overboard in the smoothie department.

Here are a few more benefits of fitting healthy energizing smoothies into your every day:

* Metabolism Boost - Weight Loss Supporter
Simply because you have control over the all-natural ingredients to put into a smoothie, you can create nutrition that is going to give your internal systems the nutrients it requires to boost your metabolism and burn fat. A well-nourished body is usually an efficient calorie burner.

You've got to eat to burn fat. Smoothies also make diversity a reality because of the limitless number of food combinations you have at your fingertips. Diversity in eating is a natural way to keep your mind and body guess-guessing, triggering more calories used and fast weight loss as a result.

Healthiest Bang for your Buck
Smoothies are an excellent way to overflow your body with nutrients and disease-fighting antioxidants that are going to help build your body strong and give you the energy to make it through the day and then some. You can also slip foods in that you might otherwise not be able to stomach. Food combinations will mask unpleasant flavors to your palate and this means you can enjoy healthy without ever suffering. The healthy raw-food combinations are endless.

Protein Plus
Protein is the key to weight loss. The idea that muscle burns more calories than fat is important when trying to lose fat and keep it off. If you build your body strong with muscle instead of fat you are going to burn more calories naturally, even when having a snooze. In order to build lean muscle you need to eat adequate amounts of lean protein on a regular basis for energy and building. If you don't your body will actually start breaking down the muscle for energy that you've already worked hard to build. This is a double loss in that you will lose some of your fat burning ability and you will burn less calories as a whole. Smoothies are a great way to ensure you are giving your body the ability to build lean muscle and burn fat fast.

Hydration
Drinking smooth and creamy smoothies will leave you hydrated and energized. Milk and yogurt in large part are water and this means you don't have to worry about the

water factor when fueling up with healthy and nutritious smoothies.

Improves Immunity - Deters Disease
By giving your body all the vital nutrients it requires on a daily basis you are building up your immunity to serious disease, flushing harmful toxins from your body that lead to disease and introducing protective mechanisms to strengthen your health further. Antioxidants from fresh berries will help to protect you, fighting those nasty free radicals that try and break down your internal systems, leaving you sick, weak and diseased.

Improves Self-Confidence
Who doesn't feel like a million bucks when they shed pounds? Losing excess baggage tends to flip your switch to positive and this will benefit your life as a whole. Stress is relieved, relations strengthened and you are much more likely to stop and smell the roses. By energizing your system and losing weight with smart smoothies you are going to set yourself up for success. Looking great and feeling better never tasted so good.

My Thoughts . . .
Smoothies can be beneficial any way you mix them. By using healthy wholesome ingredients, avoiding excess sugars, and making sure you keep an eye on the fats, you are going to gain for this fast and simple nutrient loaded beverage. In a pinch, one smoothie can give you the vitamins and minerals you may have missed out on by not having the time to cook up a meal. As with the different kinds of smoothies, the benefits truly are endless. Drink up to great health and lots of fat lost.

Where Smoothies Fit In?

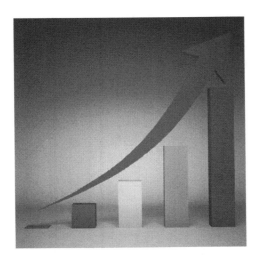

I don't care what you are talking about. Too much of a good thing isn't good. If you eat too many tasty treats you will get fat. If you try to lose fat fast with the newest whacky fad diet you will eventually gain it all back and then some, and add a little depression for bonus. If you exercise to the extreme you are eventually burn out, wear down your systems, get injured and not be able to train at all. That's just life!

Well the same applies to incorporating smoothies into your healthy lifestyle. No matter how much you LOVE them, it's important to do everything in moderation. Ease your way in and make sure you moderate because it's impossible to just survive on smoothies forever. Well, it's not impossible maybe, but let's just say impractical. Could you imagine going out for dinner with friends and having to bring your own smoothie beverage with you while everyone else eats? Silly, don't you think?

Fads come and go because they aren't sustainable. You can stick with them for a few weeks or months, until you hit your limit and then you plummet. It's important you recognize this and use smoothies positively to benefit your overall "big picture" of health.

Smoothies will help you lose weight if you use them properly if you make them with healthy, wholesome, fat-loss triggering ingredients, and drink them in moderation and ENJOY them. You need to do a little experimenting to figure out what works for you and your lifestyle, weight-loss goals, preferences, tolerances, wants and needs. If you aren't happy, then it's just not worth it, make sense?

Smoothies are excellent in curbing bad habits. Have a sweet tooth? By drinking a delicious and nutritious fruit smoothie you will give your body a nice dose of healthy sugar faster than you'd get it eating something unhealthy like a candy bar or cookie. Over time you can teach your body to crave a good sweetness instead of high-fat and nutrition-less treats. The choice is yours.

Here's how you can fit tasty and vitamin rich smoothies into your diet to lose weight fast.

* Make Breakfast a Reality
Some people just never get into the habit of eating breakfast, yet it is the most important meal of the day. Your body needs energy in order to get your physically and mentally through your day and by not eating first thing you're stressing your system, causing interference and this is just the beginning of the metabolic issues you are making. By throwing a low-fat, high-energy breakfast smoothie together fast in the morning, you are giving your body the energy it needs to burn fat and the energy to feel amazing. Why wouldn't you?

* Deter Sweet Cravings
Chances are pretty good you've got at least a little bit of a sweet tooth. Habitually eating a candy bar or nutrition-less high-fat bag of chips when your sweet cravings strike is not going to help you lose fat. It's mind over matter here.

So what's the solution?

Mix yourself a healthy nutrient dense smoothie with some fresh fruit, just enough sweetness to steer you away from your sugarless habit. With a little bit of time and a whole lot of persistence and patience you will start looking forward to your smoothie treat instead of your quick fix energy snack of unhealthy sweets. Sweet and tasty weight loss smoothies will give you the quick sweet energy you are looking for that stays in your system because of the complex carbohydrates and high energy rather than the simple carbs and loads of sugars. Makes sense, don't you think?

* Healthy Afternoon Pick-Me-Up
I don't know about you but I always seem to lose energy around 3 in the afternoon. It suddenly feels like the wind has been knocked out of my sails and my energy levels drop to rock bottom. This becomes a desperate time of weakness for most and we opt to grab an unhealthy snack to come back up to the surface. Incorporating a healthy smoothie into your afternoon instead of fast-food treat options is going to boost your fat burning enzymes, satisfy your rumbling tummy and most importantly bring your energies back up to where they belong.

* Fills You Up With Energy That Lasts
You can fuel your body with simple carbs that are "fast-fuel." Sure, they give you a quick high, but it's short-lived because soon after your energy drops and you feel like

crap. Processed and convenience packaged foods are at the brunt of it all. Smoothies will help to give your bodily systems the energy they need long-term. By incorporating a mix of lean energizing protein, complex carbohydrates and the perfect mix of fat-burning vitamins, minerals and healthy fats, a smoothie will give you the energy you need to lose weight and feel fabulous for the long run, allowing you to kiss those short lived energy bursts that screw with your blood sugars.

This also helps to decrease the risk of serious disease and illness that are connected to blood sugar fluctuation, including diabetes. Leveling your energy also helps control mood and behavior, leaving you level leaded and better able to deal with whatever life happens to throw at you.

So Easy!
This factor is just icing on the cake. Creating healthy smoothies to help you drop fat is almost too easy. All you need to do is figure out what sort of nutritious ingredients you want to use, then toss them in a blender and drink up. It really can't get much easier than that. With a little planning and practice you are going to create fantastic smoothies without even thinking about it.
In the morning on the way out the door it will just take you 5 minutes to give your body exactly what it needs to start burning fat, while leaving you with an energizing smile. It sounds all good to me.

My Thoughts . . .
The most important factor here is that you work to fit smoothies into YOUR routine. It's not about all or nothing here. It's about making smart and sustainable health choices to help you lose weight, gain energy and built your life healthy and happy. You may find that a nutritious and tasty weight loss smoothie to start your morning and

one to replace unhealthy sugar surged snacks in the afternoon works best for you, or perhaps you don't have a whole lot of time for lunch and find that a nutritious and fibrous protein smoothie works nicely for your lunch and maybe another before your head to the gym in the afternoon to give your body a nice dose of protein and staying energy to maximize your calorie burn and not deplete your energy levels completely.

I don' want you to throw in the towel here on eating real nutritious foods. I just want you to see how smoothies fit in to give your body everything it requires nutritionally and help your body burn the excess fat you want to lose weight. Perspective is important here and understanding the best thing you can do for your health and wellness is to take the information that works for you and apply it. Doing this is only going to benefit you.

Smoothie Myths De-bunked

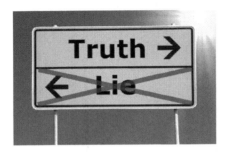

Myth - All Smoothies are Healthy
Truth - Unfortunately, refined sugars are taking the place of fruits in many commercial smoothies. These are ones that you may get while shopping or at a restaurant or cafe. Just because you are having a smoothie, don't assume it's healthy. The fact is, many smoothies have more sugar than you would get in a soda or piece of cake. The "cheaper" way to sweeten a smoothie is to give it a few pumps of corn syrup or other refined sugar. This will give you a "wallop" of extra calories and you are going to get a massive sugar rush and crash shortly after. Exactly the opposite of what a healthy fat-burning smoothie should do.

Myth - Boosted Smoothies are ALL Good
Truth - Many of the supplements used to give your smoothie a boost are modified chemically, filled with harmful synthetic ingredients. Also, take into consideration that often the quality of this "booster" and quantity is

often poor and minimal. If you look on the ingredient list it's often last to be noted. You are looking for smoothies boosted with raw organic and all-natural ingredients, ones that are readily absorbed by your body to give you the clean energy pick-me-up that does your body and mind good.

Myth - "Light" Is Always Better
Truth - Light doesn't mean healthy or better for you. Often there are chemically based sweeteners added to smoothies that are not natural and studies have shown they may cause serious health consequences over time and in large quantities. Some reported negative health implications are memory loss, headaches and fibromyalgia.

Myth - Smoothies Have Less Calories Than Soda
Lots of smoothies are loaded with high fructose corn syrup and other refined sugars that are directly linked with obesity. Be sure you know all the ingredients before drinking, particularly how it's sweetened just to be sure. Smoothies can be low-fat, low in calories and extremely nutritious, but certainly all are not.

My Thoughts . . .
If something just doesn't make sense to you then you should probably inquire further. We seem to be experts in discounting our gut feeling and accepting what we want to believe, right or wrong. By not assuming anything, paying attention to logic and most importantly asking the question, you will get the accurate information you need to make the best decisions for you and your weight loss strategy. The "right" smoothie facts are going to help you reach your weight loss goals and so much more. The "wrong" information is just going to steer you down the path toward "Frustration-Ville."

Delicious Smoothie Recipes for Energy and Weight Loss

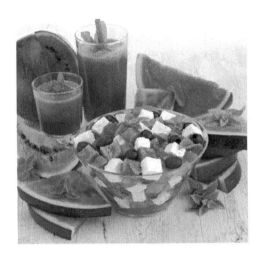

We never seem to have too much energy and of course we all want to lose at least a few pounds. Who doesn't want to look and feel better about themselves?

Here are a few delicious and nutritious Energy and Weight-Loss Smoothie recipes that will help your body get rid of excess fat and have the energy it needs to make you feel great and do all the things in life you want. Smoothies can be healthy, tasty, nutritious, and they will help you get rid of fat and replace it with limitless stores of long-term energy, but only if you're smart about it and you WANT it.

Banana Peanut Butter Smoothie
Can you say YUMMY? A smoothie that combines energy burning protein with healthy nutrients, combined with

healthy eating and regular exercise, is going to give your body what it requires to burn fat fast. Throw these tasty ingredients into the blender and get ready for a party in your mouth.

One small banana
1 tablespoon of all-natural peanut butter
1/2 cup skim milk
5 ice cubes
1 tsp chocolate whey protein powder
1 tsp flaxseed
App. 350 calories

Very Berry Smoothie
Berries are loaded with protective antioxidants that help deter disease from settling in. They also give you the energy and vitamins and minerals your system needs to function optimally, burning calories and pesky fat in the process.

One cup blueberries, blackberries, raspberries, strawberries
1/2 cup low-fat yogurt
App. 200 calories - great afternoon pick-me-up!

Strawberry and Banana Smoothie
This mixture is loaded with healthy energizing carbs and very little fat. Add to that a touch of protein and you've got the perfect tasty recipe to kick start your metabolism.

1 banana
1 cup strawberries
1/2 cup ice
1/2 low-fat milk or fat-free yogurt
App. 250 calories

Spinach Berry Smoothie
Talk about giving your day a boost! The protein, good carbs and overdose of vitamins and minerals in this beverage really will knock your socks off. Helping to

encourage your body to burn more calories and send fat a packing!
1 1/2 cups fresh baby spinach
1/2 cup light almond milk
1/2 cup fresh strawberries
1/2 cup fresh blackberries
1/2 orange
1/2 banana
1 cup ice
App. 350 calories

Zippy Veggie Sweet Smoothie
This one is a no-brainer for getting all the nutrition you need I one dose. It's an antioxidant rich, fibrous, complex carb mixture with energizing and muscle building protein, everything you need to rev up your engine and get your metabolism burning those fat cells pronto.
2 diced tomatoes
1/4 cucumber
1 tsp flaxseed
1/4 onion
1/4 tsp chili powder
1 red pepper
1/8 avocado
2 celery sticks
1/4 cups ice
1 serving egg protein
App. 350 calories

Energizer Smoothie
This smoothie will give your body and mind the energy boost it needs to perform. It's full of and minerals that will give your internal bodily functions the fuel they need to run your body optimally.
1/2 avocado
1 small apple
1/2 cup yogurt

1 cup spinach
1/2 cup blackberries
3/4 cup low-fat almond milk
App. 300 calories

Oatmeal Banana Metabolism Booster Smoothie
This is a great breakfast smooth to get you energy started right. Protein, complex carbohydrates and vitamin rich banana gives your body the energy required to blast fat and gives you a skip in your step long term.
1/2 cup non-quick cooking oatmeal
3/4 cup skim milk
1 pear
1 banana
1 tbsp flaxseed
App. 350 calories

BONUS FEATURE IMMUNITY BOOSTING SMOOTHIE
If you aren't healthy you aren't happy. Implementing a low-fat energizing Immunity Boosting Smoothie into your diet is going to help you push sickness and disease away naturally, and it takes great! It's a smoothie with Vitamin A,C, E, antioxidants, fatty acids, probiotics and zinc is going to give your system a massive dose of protection, deterring disease and injecting energy for fast use.
3 mint leaves
1/2 grapefruit
1/2 orange
1/2 cup strawberries
1/2 cup blueberries
1/2 cup raspberries
1 tsp fresh ginger
1 tsp flaxseed
1/4 tsp pure vanilla
1/4 cup pure apple juice
1/2 cup ice

Blend this tasty immune boosting smoothie up and enjoy.
App. 300 calories

My Thoughts . . .
These are a few recipes to get you started on your way to losing weight fast by adding energizing fat-burning smoothies into your diet. This strategy will help you make the right food choices and ensure your body is never nutrient deprived. Start depriving your body of essential vitamins and minerals and it will interfere with your good-health intentions.
Get creative, use the information you have gained from this book that's going to help you look great and feel fabulous, marrying your mental and physical to optimize your health.

Final Word

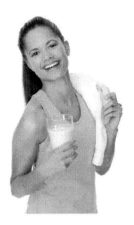

You want to know why most fat loss regimens fail? It's simply because we set ourselves up for it. We place unrealistic expectations on ourselves when eating and exercising that directly interfere with our happiness. In order to be happy you need to be content . . .
* Physically
* Mentally
* Socially
* Emotionally
* Spiritually

Each of these factors always needs attention and in order to change how you are feeling about yourself as a whole, you've got to open your mind to except and find greatness in CHANGE.

You do this by learning to make healthier eating choices in your life always, making sure you eat nutritious foods your body needs, in the right amounts and regularly, and you are going to make your body and mind function better together. Sticking with all-natural wholesome foods minus preservatives and harmful chemicals, like processed and packaged "convenience foods" have, will set you up for success in weight loss.

By incorporating nutritious, energizing, nutrient-rich and fat blasting smoothies into your diet plan each day, you're going to boost your energy, strengthen your internal systems and give fat its walking papers FAST. As humans we are impatient and want results quickly in order to actually believe the changes we are making are working. Like it or lump it that's just the way we work.

Starting your morning with a delicious energizing Breakfast Smoothie loaded with protein, good carbs and loads of micronutrients, you will kick start your metabolic processes and burn more calories than you would grabbing donut at the nearest coffee shop. That's just a lump of unhealthy saturated and Trans fat with little to ZERO nutritional value. A ticket to getting fat and feeling like crap, that likely comes in at around 350 calories, and a processed muffin is WORSE!

Your best option is to opt for the healthy, tasty, clean energy smoothie, giving you less calories and more vital energizing nutrients that will boost your energy stores up for the long run, blast fat and leave your feeling energized and alive to start your day.

A no-brainer, right?

Add to your day at least 30-45 minutes of cardiovascular exercise; hiking, biking, fast-walking, swimming, aerobic etc, and 15 minutes of weights or strength training 2-3 times a week, and you WILL be laughing your way all the way to the swimsuit shop faster than you could have ever imagined.

Is weight loss easy? It sort of can be.
Are positive lifestyle changes easy to establish for the LONG-TERM? Nope!

If you want to lose weight and keep it off for the long run you are going to need to WANT it and then you are going to have to COMMIT to sticking with it and making it happen.

Smoothies for FAST Weight Loss work. They are an important piece of good overall health. Can you lose weight and keep it off for good like many of the "Smoothie Recipe" books out there claim by just living off smoothies? NEWSFLASH ! You CAN'T!!!

It's all about tuning into the big picture. Looking at the basics of good health, the logical aspect, your preferences and tolerances and finding the FIT that works for you. Smoothies for FAST Weigh Loss will work for you by finding where in your day they fit best and plugging them in.

Don't be afraid to change things up and experiment with both the ingredients in your fat blasting smoothies but also when you have them and how much you have.

This open mind and diverse eating strategy including energizing smoothies is going to set you up to lose weight fast and keep it off long-term. You hold the cards. You are in control of you, how you perceive things and what action you take.
Ready . . . Set . . . Go!

We have the choice to look for the positive or the negative in life. You can choose to lift someone up or to stomp on them. Writing is my passion and I work hard at it, with the goal of helping make people better. If you gain a new piece of knowledge, read something that makes you think, or perhaps even smile a few times, then I am happy and content!

Life's just too short not to tune into optimism. If your glass is half full, then I invite you to read my writing, and if you have a minute to spare when you're through, **I would appreciate your review.** This will help me better myself and my writing. I thank you in advance and appreciate you.

Made in the USA
Columbia, SC
25 August 2024